Ahmed Harbaoui

Management of non-severe head injuries

Ahmed Harbaoui

Management of non-severe head injuries

The nurse's role

ScienciaScripts

Imprint

Cover image: www.ingimage.com

This book is a translation from the original published under ISBN 978-620-6-72535-0.

Publisher:
Sciencia Scripts
is a trademark of
Dodo Books Indian Ocean Ltd. and OmniScriptum S.R.L publishing group

120 High Road, East Finchley, London, N2 9ED, United Kingdom
Str. Armeneasca 28/1, office 1, Chisinau MD-2012, Republic of Moldova, Europe
Printed at: see last page
ISBN: 978-620-8-29736-7

Table of contents

INTRODUCTION

Traumatic brain injury (TBI), also known as craniocerebral trauma or cranioencephalic trauma, is a direct or indirect mechanical attack on the cranial cavity, which may cause immediate or subsequent disorders of consciousness reflecting diffuse or localized brain damage ranging from obnubilation to coma[1].

CTs vary in mechanism (blast, fall, road accident, etc.) and severity (mild to severe).

Craniocerebral damage deserves special mention and attention. Its consequences can be devastating, as lesions can be irreversible, often resulting in multiple physical impairments, cognitive impairment and behavioral problems, and detection can be delayed.

Non-severe head injuries include mild head trauma (GCS >13) and moderate head trauma 9≤GCS<13 [2].

In France, there are around 150,000 CTs per year, representing an incidence of 281/100,000 inhabitants. Of these, around 80% are mild and 11% moderate. These figures are based on the 1986 study carried out in the Aquitaine region [3].

There is a clear difference in initial somatic severity between the vulnerating organic consequences of severe CT and those of apparently benign TCL. But even if "non-severe" CT is very rarely life-threatening, some patients develop lasting complaints that contrast with the negativity of the clinical examination and the usual complementary investigations.

A good understanding of the epidemiology, pathophysiology and complications of non-severe head injuries is therefore a prerequisite for developing risk prevention campaigns (primary prevention), improving the quality of care for non-severe head injuries (secondary prevention), and managing the after-effects and socio-professional and family reintegration (tertiary prevention).

The objectives of our work are :

- Study the epidemiological, paraclinical, therapeutic and evolutionary characteristics of patients hospitalized for non-severe TC.
- Clarify the role of the nurse in the management of non-serious TC in the neurosurgical environment.

METHODS

1. Type of study

- This is a retrospective study based on a data collection sheet gathering general information on patients who have been treated for non-severe head injury, collated over a 7-year period from January 1, 2014 to December 31, 2020.

2. Study location

- Our work was carried out in the neurosurgery department of the Hôp ital Militaire Principal d'Instruction de Tunis (HMPIT).

3. Target population

- Patients admitted for non-severe head trauma to the neurosurgery department of HMPIT.

Inclusion criteria:

- o Evidence of non-severe head trauma, i.e. trauma with a Glasgow score of 15 or above.

Non-inclusion criteria :

Patient-related causes:

- o Absence of head trauma.
- o Severe head trauma.

Exclusion criteria :

- o Incomplete file
- o Running away or leaving against medical advice.

4. Data collection

- Data were collected from the medical files in the archives, using a data collection form (Appendix 1).
- The questions were grouped according to the following themes:
  - Epidemiological data: patient identity: age, sex, circumstances of head injury, admission time, length of hospital stay.
  - Clinical data: local examination, neurological examination, general examination
  - Paraclinical data: CT brain lesions
  - Therapeutic data: treatment modalities: medical/surgical
  - Evolutionary data: favorable/favorable evolution according to GSC score (Appendix 2), complications, sequelae.

5. Data analysis

- Data were entered and analyzed using Excel 2010 software.

6. Ethical and administrative considerations

- Before starting work, we requested the necessary authorization from the department head.
- The cards were all anonymous and contained no personal data.

RESULTS

Sixty-one patients (61) were admitted to the neurosurgery department of HMPIT.

I. Epidemiological data

1. Age

We classified our patients according to age into three groups (Figure 1). According to the diagram, the majority of our patients fell into the age bracket [20-50 years].

The average age of our patients was 45, with extremes ranging from 2 to 80 years.

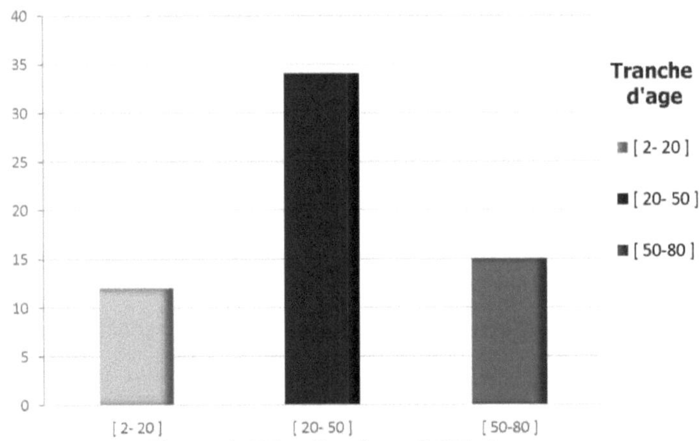

Figure 1: Distribution of CTs by age.

2. Gender

- 41 men and 20 women, with a sex ratio (male/female) of 2.05.

A clear male predominance was noted (Figure2).

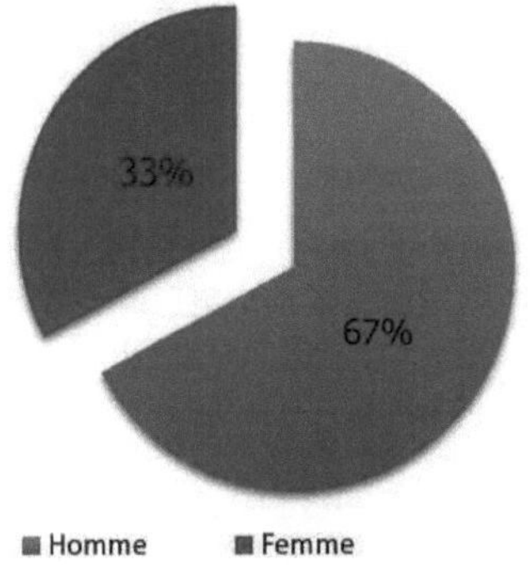

Figure 2: Distribution by gender.

3. Circumstances of head trauma

Road traffic accidents (RTAs) were the leading cause of CT in our series, with 34 patients out of the total, representing a frequency of 55.7%(Figure 3).

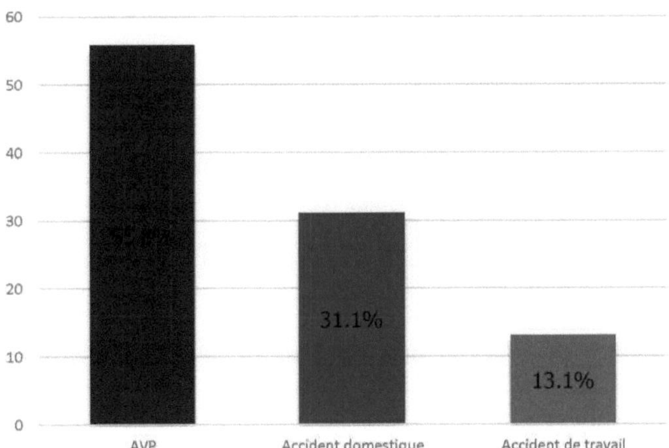

Figure 3: Distribution of CTs according to circumstances.

4. Mode of transport

It was noted that patient transport was mainly carried out by military

SMUR ambulances (Figure 4).

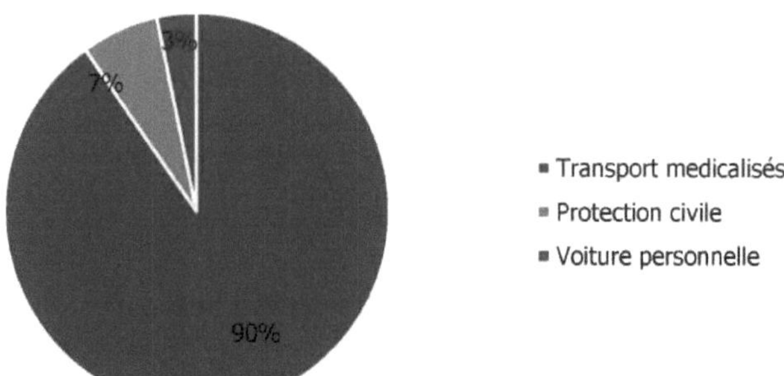

Figure 4: Medicalized/ non-medicalized transport.

5. Timeframe for care

Time to admission for head trauma patients ranged from the first 6 hours after the trauma to 24 hours (Figure 5).

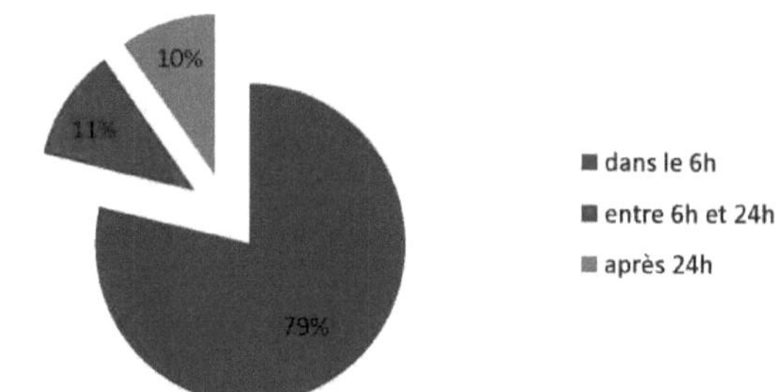

Figure 5: Distribution of CT according to time to treatment.

II. Clinical data

1. Hemodynamic status

In our series, 98.36% of patients were admitted in good general condition, with a stable hemodynamic state (Table I).

Table I: Distribution of patients according to hemodynamic status.

2. Neurological examination

HEMODYNAMIC STATUS	PERCENTAGE (%)
STABLE	98,36
INSTABLE	1,64

a. State of consciousness

In the series studied, CTs were divided into two groups according to the initial Glasgow score (Table II):

- Group 1: moderate head trauma: GCS was between 9 and 13.
- The 2nd group: mild head trauma: initial GCS was greater than or equal to 13.

Table II: Distribution of patients according to GCS.

GCS	Number	Percentage (%)
[9-13[	15	25
[13-15]	46	75

b. Deficit signs

Motor deficit was found in 5 of our patients (8.2%).

3. Other signs

They were dominated by headaches, present in 100% of cases (Figure 6).

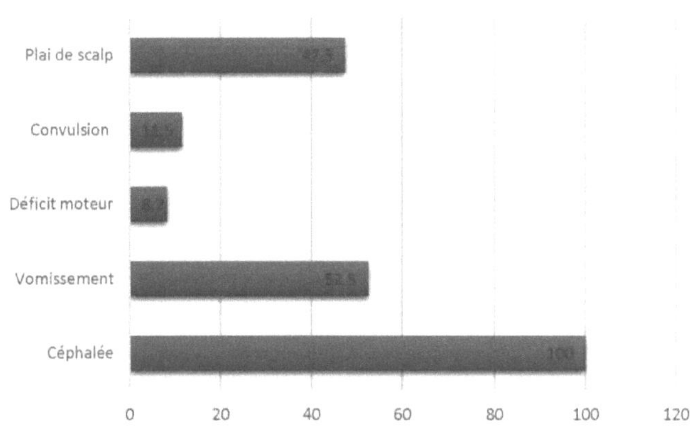

Figure 6: Distribution of patients according to clinical signs.

III. Paraclinical data

1. Brain CT

100% of patients in our series underwent emergency brain CT.

2. CT lesions

Extra-dural haematomas accounted for (50.8%), followed by embarrures (24.6%), craniocerebral wounds (16.4%) and cerebral contusions (8.2%) (Figure 7).

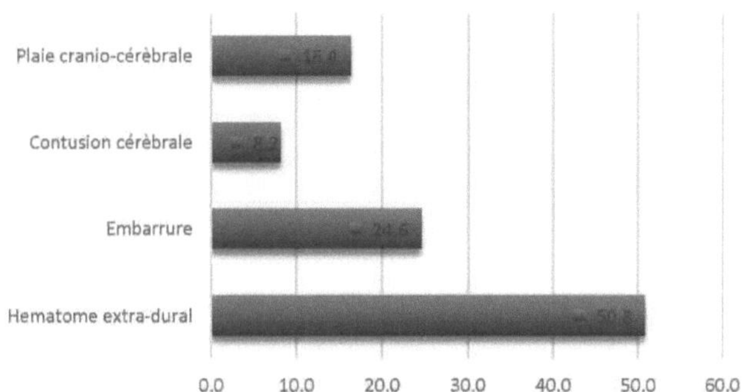

Figure 7: Distribution of patients according to CT lesions.

IV. Therapeutic data

1. Non-surgical treatment

37.7% of patients benefited from simple clinical monitoring.

2. Surgical treatment

In the series studied, 62.3% underwent surgery. (Figure 8)

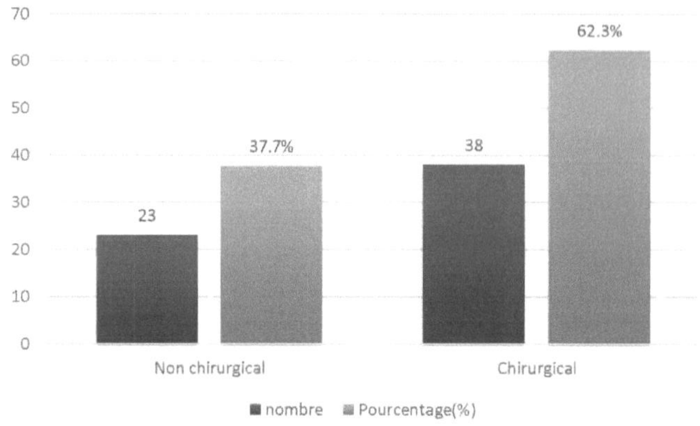

Figure 8: Distribution by therapeutic modality.

V. Evolutionary data

1. Length of hospital stay

The average duration was 5.1 days, with extremes ranging from one day to 12 days (Table III).

Table III: Distribution of patients by length of hospital stay.

Duration	Number	Percentage (%)
From 1 to 3	25	40,98
From 3 to 6	32	52,46
From 6 to 21	12	19,67

2. Evolution

A favorable outcome was observed in 58 patients.

The outcome was unfavorable in 3 patients (4.9%), including 2 cases of death from craniocerebral injury and one case of death from pulmonary embolism on day 5 of hospitalization.

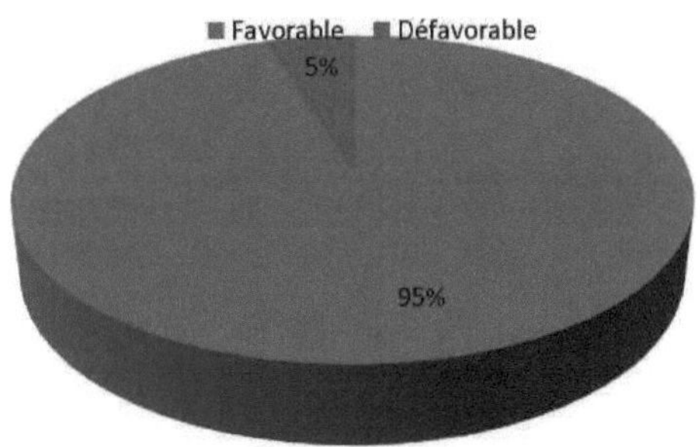

Figure 9: Distribution of patients according to their type of evolution.

3. Complications

In our series, 6 patients presented complications illustrated in Table V :

Table IV: Distribution of CTs according to complications during hospitalization.

Complication		Number	Percentages (%)
Neurological	Motor deficits	1	1,6
	Convulsion	1	1,6
Thromboembolic	Peripheral venous thrombosis	1	1,6
	Pulmonary embolism	1	1,6
Infectious	Meningitis	2	3,3

DISCUSSION

Our work consisted of a retrospective descriptive study based on a data collection form gathering general information on non-severe head injuries. Our target population consisted of a number of 61 records of patients admitted to the neurosurgery department of the Hôpital Militaire d'Instruction de Tunis from January 1, 2014 to December 31, 2020.

A. Discussion of the study

1. Highlights of our study

This work focuses on a major public health problem, due to its high frequency in most countries of the world and its socio-economic costs.

2. Weaknesses and limitations of our study

Like all scientific work, our study suffered from a number of shortcomings.

- One bias was the small number of files. A larger number could have increased the power and significance of our results.
- Inadequate information in the files also limits the quality of the data collected, but this is typical of all retrospective studies.
- Data are based on declarations by patients and/or their relatives, and on their transcription into the medical record by emergency physicians and/or neurosurgeons. This declarative mode can lead to a loss of information. In a certain number of files, for example, the time of the trauma is rarely noted in a precise manner.

  yet it is an essential element in the management of the
  charge.

Results analysis

I. Epidemiology

1. **Age distribution**

Most studies show an average age of between 30 and 50 years [4] . According to Stnik et al. the median age in the United States is 40, with a distribution of peaks at 17 and 44 years of age[4].

In our study, the average age of the population studied was 45, with extremes ranging from 2 to 80 years, which is in line with the literature. The high frequency of cases in this age group could be explained by the high level of physical and, above all, professional activity at this time of life.

2. **Breakdown by gender**

Most studies of CT show a male predominance, with a sex ratio generally greater than 2.

In our series, there was a male predominance, with a sex ratio of 2.05. This may be explained by the fact that men are more exposed to the various etiological factors of CT (MVA, aggression, falls, etc.).

Table V: Comparison of sex ratios in different studies.

Various studies	Country of origin	Sex ratio
Our study	**Tunisia**	**2,05**
HADDAR et al [5]	**Marrakech**	**4,08**
TALEB et al [6]	**Algeria**	**4,46**
Stnik et al [4]	**United States**	**1.10**

II. Etiology

1. Road accidents (AVP)

According to most studies, MVAs are the main cause of head trauma [2]. According to Masson et al, MVAs are the leading cause of head trauma, accounting for 48.3%[2]. In fact, they are the leading cause of morbidity in developed countries.

In our study, MVAs were the leading cause of trauma, accounting for 55.7%.

The mortality and morbidity caused by road accidents should prompt the authorities to think more carefully about the subject. A strict regime such as speed limits and tighter controls, alcohol testing and seat belts can undeniably bring about a clear reduction in the morbidity and mortality of MVAs.

2. Domestic accidents

According to a study by TALEB et al, domestic accidents account for 23.3% of cases[6].

In our series, the frequency of domestic accidents was 31.1%.

3. Work-related accidents

According to WAKRIM et al [8], the frequency of work-related accidents is 1.9%, lower than the 13.1% we found.

Some professions require considerable physical effort. What's more, assembly-line work, involving the repetition of the same movement, increases the risk of accidents by reducing concentration.

4. Transport arrangements

According to the study by TALEB et al, more than half of all CT cases (53%) did not receive medical transport from the accident site to a medical facility or university hospital[6].

In our series, 90% of our patients benefited from medical transport, compared with 10% from non-medical transport.

Indeed, the creation of the military SAMU in 2013 has led to a radical transformation in the first aid administered, as well as a frankly significant improvement in the quality of emergency care for patients and their prognosis.

5. Timeframe for care

According to the study by FATMA et al, around 85% of patients consult within 6 hours of the trauma, which is in line with our study (around 79% of our patients consulted within the first 6 hours)[5].

According to the study by TALEB et al., 30% of TC were even admitted to hospital within 3 hours of the accident [6].

This is one of the elements most closely correlated with the prognosis of traumatic brain injuries.

III. Clinical data

1. Hemodynamic status

Correction of hypotension is a standard part of neurosurgical resuscitation. Hypotension is described as systolic blood pressure <90 mm Hg. It is essential to correct any hypotension, as it increases the risk of secondary cerebral aggression and increases mortality, particularly if associated with hypoxia.

In our series, 98.36% of patients were admitted in good general condition, with a stable hemodynamic state.

2. **Neurological condition**

We can determine the degree of severity of CT using clinical scales. The most widely used is the Glasgow Coma Scale (Appendix 2), which examines the three types of clinical response to conventional stimuli: eye opening, verbal response, motor response.

Generally speaking, three degrees of severity are recognized: severe, moderate and mild traumatic brain injury [9]. Non-severe head injuries therefore include moderate and mild head injuries.

A Glasgow score between 13 and 15, when assessed 30 minutes or more after the accident, defines mild TC. These manifestations must not be due to alcohol or other drug intoxication; nor must they be caused by a treatment implemented in the initial phase of the trauma.

11 may be associated with a period of altered consciousness (confusion, disorientation) or loss of consciousness lasting less than 30 minutes, or post-traumatic amnesia lasting less than 24 hours, or any other transient neurological sign such as a localized neurological sign, convulsion or intracranial lesion not requiring surgical intervention.

Internationally, the differences in the definition of mild head injury concern loss of consciousness, which is sometimes limited to 15 minutes, and post-traumatic amnesia, which may be limited to 30 minutes. Moderate cranial trauma corresponds to a Glasgow score between 9 and 12 which may be associated with a loss of consciousness ranging from 30 minutes to 6 hours, and post-traumatic amnesia between 24 hours and 14 days. Other studies suggest a loss of consciousness from 15 minutes to 6 hours, and post-traumatic amnesia between 30 minutes and 24 hours, with the possibility of a skull fracture but no underlying brain injury.

According to the Société Française de Neurochirurgie, severe head trauma is defined by a Glasgow score of 8 or less.

In our study, all CTs were non-severe, with 75% of initial GCSs greater than or equal to 13.

IV. Paraclinical data

1. Brain CT

Cerebral CT can be used to establish emergency neurosurgical indications, particularly when there is clear compression of the cerebral parenchyma and medial structures **[11]**.

In our series, 100% of patients benefited from brain CT.

2. CT lesions

- Extradural hematoma (EHD)

It results from the formation of a blood collection between the cranium and dura mater, and is most often associated with a skull fracture. It results from damage to a meningeal artery or vein, or more rarely from rupture of a venous sinus. Diagnosed by CT scan, it presents as a spontaneously hyperdense, well-limited, biconvex lens, with a mass effect on the adjacent parenchyma**[12]**.

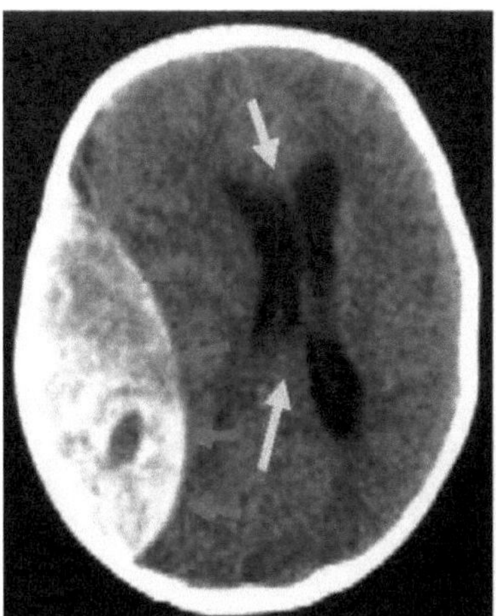

Figure 10: Cerebral CT scan showing an extradural hematoma.

In our series, HED was present in half the cases (50.8%).

- **Cerebral contusion**

Hemorrhagic contusions are areas of cerebral destruction resulting from the direct impact of the brain against protruding parts of the cranial bone structure. For this reason, they most often occur in the frontal and temporal lobes. Hemorrhagic contusions consist of a hyperdense, hemorrhagic central core surrounded by an area of hypodense, hypoperfused brain tissue at risk of ischemia. In the hours and days following the trauma, a pericontusional edematous halo forms, with ischemic (cytotoxic) and vasogenic mechanisms **[12]**.

In our series, cerebral contusions were 8.2%.

- **Lock**

This is a fracture of the skull, with the fractured part of the skull being pushed in. It causes compression of the underlying brain region, often resulting in local hemorrhage between the bone and the meninges (extradural hematoma) **[13]**.

In our series, embarrure was present in 24.6% of cases.

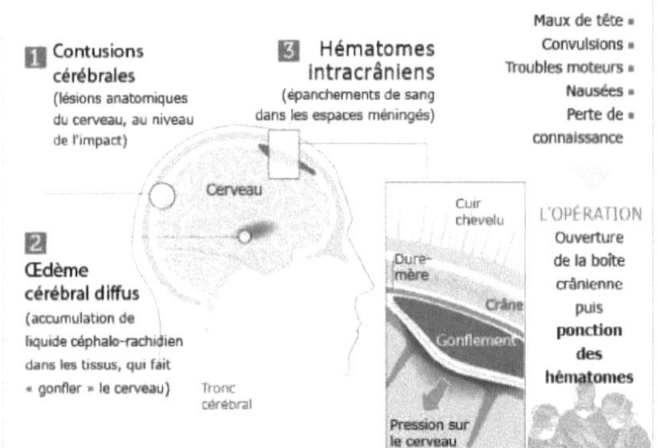

Figure 11: Possible consequences of head trauma.

V. Therapeutic data

1. Monitoring procedures

For all patients admitted for observation for non-severe CT, the observational data are: GCS, pupil size and reactivity, limb motricity, respiratory rate, heart rate, blood pressure, temperature, blood oxygen saturation. These data should be collected and recorded every half-hour until GCS reaches 15. The minimum frequency of monitoring for patients with a GCS of 15 should be as follows, commencing after initial assessment in the emergency department: every half-hour for two hours, then every hour for four hours, then every two hours. If a patient with a GCS of 15 deteriorates at any time after the initial two-hour period, monitoring should resume every half-hour and follow the initial program. **[14]**

If the head injury is minor and causes no symptoms other than pain at the site of injury, a mild analgesic such as paracetamol can be used.

Aspirin and other non-steroidal anti-inflammatory drugs should not be taken, as they can aggravate any bleeding in the brain or skull. Doctors stitch or use medical staples to close scalp wounds and then apply dressings or bandages. **[15]**

2. Surgical treatment

Surgical treatment was used in 38 cases (37.7%) and consisted of :

- Trimming of scalp wounds.
- Removal of bone splinters and foreign bodies in the case of craniocerebral wounds or embarrure, with dural repair if necessary.
- Cleansing of the cerebral focus with saline detersion of the dilated area.
- Evacuation of any intracranial hematoma in the event of acute extra- or subdural hematoma.
- Pre- and post-operative antibiotic therapy.

➢ All patients underwent surgery under general anaesthetic.

VI. Scalable data

1. Length of hospital stay

The 2005 ORS study [16] on TC (whatever the degree of severity) found hospital stays ranging from 1 day to 32 months, with an average length of 2 months. Rehabilitation lasts an average of 3.3 months, with a minimum of 11 days and a maximum of 42 months.

In our study, it averaged 5.1 days, with extremes ranging from one day to 12 days.

2. GOS classification

The Glasgow Outcome Scale (GOS) is the scale commonly used to classify the disability of a CT patient. Created in 1975 by Jennet and Bond, it was designed as a prognostic scale [17]. It comprises 5 groups based on the patient's state of consciousness, degree of dependence, and social and professional life. A new version was published in 1998: the Glasgow Outcome Scale Extended (GOSE), which includes 8 possible scores instead of 5 [18], making it possible to systematize outcome classes in terms of mortality, functional outcome and economic reintegration of the injured person (Appendix 4).

3. After-effects

The sequellar state is defined as a residual pathological state that no treatment is capable of changing. Its importance for socio-professional reintegration depends on the type of sequelae. We can state that these sequelae are numerous, ranging from mild to severe, and may manifest themselves in one or more of the following dimensions:

- The physical dimension
- The cognitive dimension
- The psycho-affective dimension
- The socio-behavioral dimension

➢ Physical dimension

The picture is one of headache, motor deficit, vegetative state and epilepsy, occurring early in adults or late after several months or even years.

➢ . Cognitive dimension

- Memory and learning disorders. The literature shows that memory is the cognitive activity most altered by CT.

- Attention deficit: like any brain injury, CT is accompanied by an attention deficit due to cognitive fatigue and slowness in processing information.
- Spoken and written language disorders; these can be at different levels (comprehension disorders, dysarthria, dyslexia, dysgraphia), afferent (perception and comprehension) and/or efferent (expression).

➢ Psycho-affective dimension

- Anxiety-depressive disorders with reduced initiative and motivation
- Poorly controlled euphoria and impulsivity, emotional lability
- Lifting of inhibitions and excessive familiarity (may be part of a frontal syndrome)
- Prioritizing primary needs
- Post-traumatic hysteria or neurosis
- Hallucinations
- Change in self-image, depersonalization, devaluation, guilt, inability to fulfill roles (family or other)

➢ Sociobehavioral dimension :

- Reduced intellectual autonomy
- Interruption of school or work activities

Special case: Subjective post-concussion syndrome :

The so-called "subjective syndrome" of head injury occurs most often after moderate head trauma. It is characterized by a protracted course, lasting months or even years. It manifests itself in anxiety, dizziness, headaches, intolerance to noise and crowds, difficulty in intellectual concentration, and a certain degree of affective regression.

Considered for a long time as a set of functional manifestations, it would seem in fact that these disorders are underpinned by undeniable organic lesions, which modern means of exploration are unable to objectify [19].

VII. Nursing role

1. Role of the Reception and Orientation Nurse (IAO)

Any patient presenting to an ED with CT must be assessed by the IOA and/or emergency physician within 15 minutes of arrival at the hospital. Prioritization of care will be defined by a triage scale. With all the information gathered, the IOA will be able to assign a degree of urgency to the patient. Here are the criteria for patient referral, based on the Canadian Triage & Acuity Scale for Emergency Departments.

Degré 1 (Installation immédiate)	Traumatisme crânien avec score de Glasgow inférieur à 10
Degré 2 (Evaluation médicale dans les 15 mn)	Traumatisme crânien avec Glasgow inférieur à 13 Céphalées intenses Perte de conscience Confusion Cervicalgies Nausées/ Vomissements Assaut avec un objet contendant autre que le poing ou les pieds. Chute de > 3 pieds ou 5 marches Piéton heurté par un véhicule Accident de voiture : éjection du véhicule, passager non attaché s'étant heurté la tête contre le pare-brise.
Degré 3 (Evaluation médicale dans les 30 mn)	Traumatisme crânien avec Glasgow à 14-15 Douleur modérée inférieur à 8/10 Nausées/ Vomissements Chute ou trébuchement en marchant sur le sol Accident de voiture : faible impact (< 30 km/h) et conducteur attaché Bataille à poings fermés ou coup à la tête (excluant avec objet pointu ou lourd) sans perte de conscience

Figure 12: Canadian Triage & Severity Scale.

2. Pre-hospital care

In our series, patients were mainly transported by ambulance. Patients benefited from essential care, notably stabilization of the cervical spine in a neck brace, with strict adherence to cervical spine alignment, and compression dressings to ensure hemostasis in the event of a wound.

3. Care in the neurosurgery department

On admission

Nursing care :

- Settling the patient in bed.
- Monitoring including heart rate and respiratory rate
- Measuring blood pressure
- Pulse oxygen saturation monitoring (Spo2) and hourly diuresis.
- Two peripheral venous lines taken.
- Complete check-up on medical prescription
- Treatment of associated lesions: suture of a hemorrhagic scalp wound.
- Stabilization of hemodynamic status and, if necessary, use of vasoactive drugs.
- Additional paraclinical workup.

Consciousness monitoring

Psychological support :

- Listening to the patient
- Explain therapeutic modalities

Post-operative

✓ Neurological monitoring :

- The state of consciousness
- Signs of HTIC: headache, vomiting and visual disturbances

✓ Hemodynamic monitoring :

- Pulse
- Blood pressure

✓ Respiratory monitoring :

- Respiratory frequency
- O2 saturation

✓ Temperature monitoring.

✓ Diuresis monitoring.

✓ Blood glucose monitoring.

✓ Pain monitoring: to adapt analgesic treatment and have it modified by the doctor if necessary.

✓ Dressing change: to prevent infection or clot formation, protect the wound, aid healing and ensure patient comfort and hygiene.

- According to medical prescription (generally every 48 hours)
- Maintain rigorous asepsis
- The dressing must be occlusive, sterile and always clean.

✓ Monitor the condition of the surgical wound:

- Cleanliness
- Bank disunion
- Inflammatory aspect

✓ Monitoring complications related to decubitus :

- Change position to prevent pressure sores and monitor head position to avoid pressure on the craniectomy area.
- Ensure nutritional balance.

✓ Biological monitoring: on medical prescription.

Nursing care :

- Toilet help for certain patients.
- Bed repair, bed hygiene.

4. **Education for the return home**

Patient discharge must be well prepared and personalized. All patients with non-severe CT deemed fit for discharge should receive written discharge recommendations (Appendix 5)[14]. Hence the role of patient education concerning complications and advice on rapid recovery. (brochure)

VII. Recommendations

With the aim of improving the management of non-severe head trauma patients, we propose a model monitoring form. By involving the paramedical staff more closely, this could certainly improve the quality of nursing supervision in this type of patient, and thus better detect in time any kind of complication requiring urgent intervention by the attending physician.

As a result, once approved by the department head, this template could be adopted into daily practice in the neurosurgery department of the Hôpital Militaire Principal d'Instruction de Tunis, making the nursing staff more active and involved in their supervisory role. **(Appendix 3)**

PREVENTION

Preventing MVAs as the primary cause of accidents is a major concern in our country. There are three complementary aspects to prevention:

-Primary prevention: aims to avoid accidents by complying with traffic rules, in order to drastically reduce the "road threat".

-tertiary prevention: aims to optimize care for accident victims and their after-effects.

Measures appropriate to each of these times include incentive actions (education campaigns, for example), authoritative actions of a legislative or regulatory type, the development by car manufacturers of passive protection against the mechanical forces at play in the trauma, and improvements in pick-up and first-aid conditions, aimed at shortening response times.[10].

CONCLUSIONS

It is within the framework of a theoretical and practical study carried out at the Hôpital Militaire Principal d'Instruction du Tunis, and more specifically in the neurosurgery department, that the present work takes place. Its theme is the role of the nurse in the management of non-severe head injuries.

This hospital-based study looked at the different therapeutic modalities for non-severe head injuries, and clarified the nursing role in the management of this pathology.

Traumatic brain injury (TBI) is a common condition, most often affecting adult males, and is mainly caused by road accidents. The impact on brain function varies in severity according to the extent of the injury.

The nurse is one of the pillars of the multidisciplinary management of this pathology. It is the nurse who initially takes charge of the patient on admission. In addition to carrying out the medical team's prescriptions, they are also responsible for the clinical monitoring of these patients. He or she must master the specific gestures and attitudes required for quality care in the neurosurgery department, while not neglecting psychological care, explanations and support for the patient's family and relatives.

In view of the importance of monitoring in the management of non-severe head injuries, and based on our findings and the literature search carried out, we have proposed a 24-hour monitoring form for these patients.

REFERENCES

[1] E. Masson, "Intracranial hypertension", *EM-Consulte,* Apr. 21, 2021. https://www.em- consulte.com/article/2373/intracranial-hypertension (accessed Apr. 21, 2021).

[2] E. Jehle, "Mild head trauma", p. 10.

[3] L. Tiret *et al,* "The epidemiology of head trauma in Aquitaine (France), 1986: a communitybased study of hospital admissions and deaths", *Int. J. Epidemiol,* vol. 19, n° 1, Art. n° 1, March 1990, doi: 10.1093/ije/19.1.133.

[4] L. Setnik and J. Bazarian, "The characteristics of patients who do not seek medical treatment for traumatic brain injury," *Brain Inj. BI,* vol. 21, pp. 1-9, Feb. 2007, doi: 10.1080/02699050601111419.

[5] "these206-16.pdf". Accessed: May 14, 2021. [Online]. Available at: http://wd.fmpm.uca.ma/biblio/theses/annee-htm/FT/2016/these206-16.pdf

[6] "PRISE-EN-CHARGE-ET-DEVENIR-DES-TRAUMATISES-CRANIENS-HOSPITALISES-AU-CHU-DE-TLEMCEN-EN-2009-ET-2010.pdf". Accessed: May 12, 2021. [Online]. Available at: http://dspace.univ-tlemcen.dz/bitstream/112/5028/1/PRISE- EN-CHARGE-ET-DEVENIR-DES-TRAUMATISES-CRANIENS-HOSPITALISES-AU-DE-TLEMCEN-EN-2009-ET-2010.pdf

[7] F. Masson *et al,* "Epidemiology of Severe Brain Injuries: A Prospective Population-Based Study", *J. Trauma Acute Care Surg,* vol. 51, n° 3, pp. 481-489, Sept. 2001.

[8] "these11-10.pdf". Accessed: May 05, 2021. [Online]. Available at: http://wd.fmpm.uca.ma/biblio/theses/annee-htm/FT/2010/these11-10.pdf

[9] L. Kosakevitch-Ricbourg, "Méthodes d'étude clinique des traumatismes crâniens", *Rev. Stomatol. Chir. Maxillofac.* vol. 107, n° 4, pp. 211-217, Sept. 2006, doi: 10.1016/S0035- 1768(06)77043-7.

[10] "orientations_traumatisme.pdf". Accessed: May 11, 2021. [Online]. Available at: https://publications.msss.gouv.qc.ca/msss/fichiers/2006/orientations_traumatisme.pdf

[11] "jpmiss2.free.fr/Divers/SFAR_2006/ca00/html/ca00_24/00_24.htm". Accessed: May 11, 2021. [Online]. Available from: http://jpmiss2.free.fr/Divers/SFAR_2006/ca00/html/ca00_24/00_24.htm

[12] V. Degos, T. Lescot, L. Abdennour, A. L. Boch, and L. Puybasset, "Surveillance et réanimation des traumatisés crâniens graves", *EMC - Anesth.-Réanimation*, vol. 4, n° 2, p. 1-20, Jan. 2007, doi: 10.1016/S0246-0289(07)44755-7.

[13] É. Larousse, "embarrure - LAROUSSE".

https://www.larousse.fr/encyclopedie/medical/embarrure/12732 (accessed May 11, 2021).

[14] steering committee *et al,* "Traumatisme crânien léger (score de Glasgow de 13 à 15) : triage, évaluation, examens complémentaires et prise en charge précoce chez le nouveau-né, l'enfant et l'adulte: Société française de médecine d'urgence", *Ann. Fr. Médecine Urgence,* vol. 2, n° 3, pp. 199-214, May 2012, doi: 10.1007/s13341-012-0202-4.

[15] "Presentation of head injuries - Injuries and intoxications", *MSD manuals for the general public.* https://www.merckmanuals.com/fr-ca/accueil/l%C3%A9sions-et-intoxications/trauma-cr%C3%A2niens/pr%C3%A9sentation-des-traumatismes-cr%C3%A2niens (accessed May 14, 2021).

[16] Yumpu.com, "consquences familiales, sociales et professionnelles - Handiplace", *yumpu.com.* https://www.yumpu.com/fr/document/read/48316907/consacquences-familiales-social-and-professional-handiplace (accessed May 12, 2021).

[17] B. Jennett and M. Bond, "ASSESSMENT OF OUTCOME AFTER SEVERE BRAIN DAMAGE: A Practical Scale", *The Lancet,* vol. 305, n° 7905, pp. 480-484, March 1975, doi: 10.1016/S0140-6736(75)92830-5.

[18] J. T. L. Wilson, L. E. L. Pettigrew, and G. M. Teasdale, "Structured Interviews for the Glasgow Outcome Scale and the Extended Glasgow Outcome Scale: Guidelines for Their Use," *J. Neurotrauma,* vol. 15, n° 8, pp. 573-585, August 1998, doi: 10.1089/neu. 1998.15.573.

[19] Doctissimo, "Post-concussion syndrome - Definition of post-concussion syndrome
concussion", *Doctissimo.* https://www.doctissimo.fr/sante/dictionnaire-medical/syndrome-post-commotionnel (accessed May 14, 2021).

APPENDICES

Annexe 1 : fiche d'exploration

Identité:

Nom et prénom :...

Age :......................................

Sexe : ○ H ○ F

ATCD : ○Oui :...○ RAS

Circonstance :

Date et heure : ....

Accident de travail ○

Accident domestique ○

Agression : Pierre Arme blanche bâton Autre:............

AVP :

-Lieu : ○ Urbain ○ Rural

-Route : ○Rue○ Route○Route nationale Autoroute○ Piste ○

-Victime : Nombre ....,dont............. décès

-type :

Piéton:

Motocycliste: casqué: oui ○ non ○

Voiture : ceinturé: oui ○ non ○

Poids lourd : ceinturé: oui ○ non ○

-Impact : ○ Frontal ○ Latéral ○ arrière

Transport:

-Délai : ○ 3H ○ 3H -6H ○ >6H

-Mode : ○ SMUR ○ Pompier ○ Ambulance ○ Témoins

-Médicalisé : ○ Oui ○ Non

Examen à l'admission :

Hémodynamique:

TA:..............mm hg FC:..............bpm

Hémorragie:

○ Exteriorisé: ○ Epistaxis ○ Otorragie ○Hémoptysie ○Plaie Autre..........

○ Interne:..

○ Pas d'hémorragie

Neurologique :

Score de Glasgow : ..../15

Pupilles: ○ Normales ○ Aniosocorie(coté:........)

○ Mydriase bilatéral : ○ Réactive ○ Areactive

Déficit neurologique: ○ Non ○ Oui Type:....................

Plaie de scalp: ○ Oui ○ Non

Embarrure : ○ Oui ○ Non

Examen des membres :

Impotence fonctionnelle : ○ Présente :siége .... ○ RAS

Déformation : ○ RAS ○ Bras ○ Avant br ○ Ma ○ Cuis ○ Jam ○ pied

Douleur : ○ RAS ○ Bra ○ Avant b ○ M ○ Cu ○ Jan ○ pied

Autre :...

Bilan radiologique :

TDM cérébrale	Oui ○	Non ○
TDM cérébrale de contrôle	Oui ○	Non ○
Rx rachis cervical	Oui ○	No ○
Rx thorax	Ou ○	No ○
Echo abdominale	Oui ○	No ○
Rx des membres	Oui ○	Non ○

Bilan biologique :

NFS	Oui ○	Non ○
VS/CRP	Ou ○	Non ○
Hémostase	Oui ○	Non ○
Ionogramme	Oui ○	Non ○

Prise en charge thérapeutique :

Antalgique : ○ Oui ○ Non Si oui : Molécule:...............

Antibiotique : ○ Oui ○ Non Si oui : Molécule:...............

Prévention du tétanos : ○ Oui ○ Non

Autres traitements : ....

Evolution :

-A court terme : Favorable

Défavorable: -HTIC: oui non ○ ○

-Infection nosocomiale oui non ○ ○

-Escarres oui non ○ ○

Autre :...

→ **GCS** à la sortie : ....

-A moyen terme:

→**GCS** à j28 du traumatisme : ....

-A long terme :

→Séquelles : ....

Appendix 2: Glasgow Coma Scale (GCS)

Enfant/Adulte		
Activité	**Score**	**Description**
Ouverture des yeux	4	Spontanée
	3	À la demande
	2	À la douleur
	1	Aucune
Réponse verbale	5	Orientée
	4	Confuse
	3	Paroles inappropriées
	2	Sons incompréhensibles
	1	Aucune
Réponse motrice	6	Obéit aux commandes
	5	Localise à la douleur
	4	Retrait à la douleur
	3	Flexion anormale (décortication)
	2	Extension anormale (décérébration)
	1	Aucune

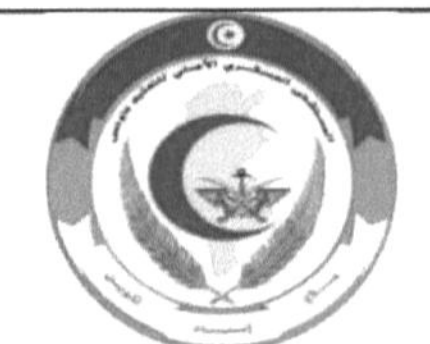	Hôpital Militaire Principal d'Instruction de Tunis
	Fiche de surveillance pendant 24h

First and last name: Personnel number:

24-hour monitoring chart														Date :										
Time	**8**	**9**	**10**	**11**	**12**	**13**	**14**	**15**	**16**	**17**	**18**	**19**	**20**	**21**	**22**	**23**	**24**	**1**	**2**	**3**	**4**	**5**	**6**	**7**
Awareness																								
Mental state																								
Drug treatment																								
Pulse																								
TA																								
Temperature																								
Oxygen saturation																								
Respiratory frequency																								
Power supply																								
Hydration																								
Intestinal elimination																								
Urinary elimination																								
Toiletries/body hygiene																								

Safety isolation area																								
Another parameter:																								

Appendix 3: 24h monitoring form

Appendix 4: GOS classification

Score ♦	Détail ♦
1	Décés
2	**Etat végétatif persistant** (Absence d'activité corticale)
3	**Handicap sévère** (Conscient mais dépendant : atteinte mentale ou motrice ou les deux)
4	**Handicap modéré**. Patient cependant autonome dans la vie quotidienne (dysphasie, hémiparésie, ataxie, troubles intellectuels ou de mémoire, troubles de la personnalité)
5	**Bonne récupération** Activités normales (déficits neurologiques ou psychologiques mineurs)

Appendix 5: Exit recommendations

Malades âgés de plus de 12 ans

Nous pensons que vous pouvez maintenant quitter l'hôpital. Après votre retour à domicile, il est peu probable que vous ayez des problèmes.

Mais si un quelconque des symptômes suivants (ré)apparaissait, il conviendrait de revenir rapidement (ou de vous faire conduire) vers la structure d'urgence la plus proche :

- *perte de connaissance ou baisse de vigilance (difficultés à garder les yeux ouverts) ;*
- *état confusionnel (désorientation, faire des choses incohérentes) ;*
- *somnolence inhabituelle ;*
- *troubles de la compréhension ou de la parole ;*
- *trouble de l'équilibre ou difficulté à la marche ;*
- *faiblesse d'un ou plusieurs membres ;*
- *problème de vision ;*
- *céphalée importante progressive, résistante ;*
- *vomissement, nausée ;*
- *convulsion (perte de connaissance, malaise) ;*
- *écoulement par le nez ou les oreilles ;*
- *saignement de l'oreille ;*
- *diminution d'acuité auditive uni- ou bilatérale.*

Éléments qui ne doivent pas vous inquiéter

Vous pouvez présenter certains symptômes dans les prochains jours qui doivent disparaître dans les 15 jours suivants. Par exemple : mal de tête modéré, nausée (sans vomissement), vertige, irritabilité ou trouble de l'humeur, difficulté de concentration ou problèmes de mémoire, fatigue, manque d'appétit, troubles du sommeil.

Si ces signes ne disparaissaient pas après deux semaines, vous devez consulter votre médecin. Nous vous conseillons également de prendre conseil auprès d'un médecin pour votre aptitude à conduire un véhicule automobile ou un deux roues.

Conseils vous permettant d'aller mieux

Les conseils suivants vont vous permettre d'aller mieux et de faire disparaître plus rapidement certains signes :

- *ne restez pas seul à domicile au cours des 48 heures après la sortie de l'hôpital ;*
- *assurez-vous que vous pouvez atteindre facilement un téléphone et appeler un médecin ;*
- *restez au calme et évitez les situations de stress ;*
- *ne prenez pas d'alcool ni de médicaments ;*
- *ne prenez pas de somnifères, sédatifs, tranquillisants, sans avis médical ;*
- *ne pratiquez pas de sport de contact (rugby, football...) pendant au moins trois semaines sans en avoir parlé à un médecin ;*
- *ne retournez pas à l'école, au collège ou à votre travail si vous n'avez pas totalement récupéré ;*
- *ne conduisez pas de voiture ni de véhicules à deux roues ni d'engin mécanique tant que la récupération n'est pas complète.*

N° de téléphone de l'hôpital : ....

Après (plus tard)

La majorité des malades récupèrent rapidement après leur accident et ne présentent aucun problème ultérieurement. Cependant, certains patients peuvent présenter quelques difficultés après quelques semaines ou mois. Si vous commencez à ressentir ces difficultés (trouble de mémoire, sensation de mal-être), contactez votre médecin dès que possible.

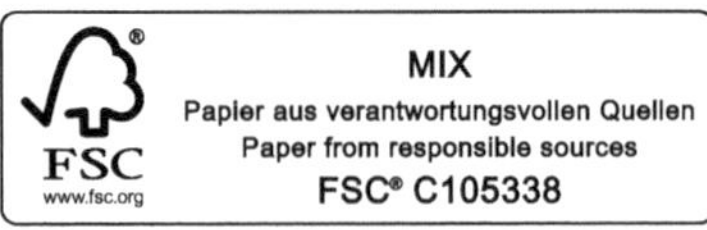

Printed by Books on Demand GmbH, Norderstedt / Germany